ROZA KAY

Healthy Aging

A Practical Guide to Living Your Best Life, Every Decade

Contents

1

Chapter 1: The Biology of Aging: Dispelling Myths and Discovering Facts

Aging. It's a term that brings to mind wrinkles, gray hair, and aching joints. But what exactly is aging? Is it just the passage of time, a never-ending march towards decay? Is there anything more complicated at work?

In this chapter, we'll delve into the fascinating realm of aging biology, dispelling misconceptions and uncovering the complicated dance of cells, genes, and environment that determines our journey through time.

Myth #1: Aging is just a matter of wearing out

Consider your body to be an automobile. Parts wear down with each mile driven, performance deteriorates, and it finally sputters to a standstill. This is a common comparison used to describe aging, however it is much too basic. Our bodies are complex ecosystems teeming with billions of cells that are continuously regenerating and adapting. While some wear and tear is unavoidable, aging involves more than just running out of spare parts.

Truth 1: Aging is a Complicated Orchestration

Consider aging to be a symphony, with several instruments (genes, proteins, and biological processes) playing in unison. The speed may shift over time, certain instruments may become less efficient, and new melodies may arise. However, the orchestra does not cease playing; rather, it finds new methods to express itself.

Our DNA, the blueprint for life, is a vital part of this symphony. Genes that control everything from hair color to longevity are found inside its double helix. Some genes, such as the well-known telomeres at the ends of chromosomes, shorten with each cell division and may play a role in aging. However, genes do not determine fate. The environment conducts the music, regulating gene expression and defining our aging trajectory via factors such as nutrition, exercise, and stress.

Myth #2: We all age at the same rate

Have you ever noticed how some individuals look to age gracefully, but others appear to be much older than their years? This is because aging is not a one-size-fits-all process. The pace of our unique symphonies is influenced by genetics, lifestyle choices, and even chance. Some individuals are inclined to live longer lives, while others confront genetic problems that may hasten some elements of aging.

Truth #2: Your Decisions Count

The good news is that we're not just passing through on this adventure. To some degree, we can affect the music. While we cannot modify our DNA, we may influence our surroundings. A nutritious diet rich in fruits, vegetables, and whole grains fuels the orchestra. Regular physical activity keeps the instruments supple and in tune. Stress management contributes to the symphony's harmony. These decisions do not ensure perpetual youth, but they may have a major influence on our healthspan, or the number of years we live free of chronic illnesses and disabilities.

Exploring Aging Research Frontiers

The science of aging biology is always changing, revealing new mysteries and promising treatments. Scientists are looking at the potential of:

Telomere Repair: Could we develop methods to prolong or preserve telomeres, possibly reducing cellular aging?

Senescence Reversal: Can dormant cells be reactivated to renew tissues and organs?

Epigenetic reprogramming: Can we change how genes are expressed to alter aging?

While many of these topics remain unsolved, the potential is exciting. Aging's future may not be about halting time, but rather about learning to direct our symphonies with more ability and awareness.

Remember that aging is a tale, not a sentence. We've begun to examine the first few chapters of that tale in this chapter, diving into the myths and reality of our biological journey. Let us have an open mind as we go ahead, enjoy the complexity, and uncover the melody that makes our symphonies of aging wonderfully beautiful.**

An In-Depth Look at Aging Theories:

Theory of Free Radicals: According to this common idea, aging is caused by a buildup of free radicals, which are reactive chemicals that harm cells and DNA. Consider them to be microscopic vandals causing havoc in your cellular metropolis. Antioxidants, which may be found in fruits and vegetables, serve as city watchmen, neutralizing free radicals and defending your cellular architecture. While the importance of free radicals cannot be overstated, there is more to the picture. Inflammation and metabolic abnormalities are two more elements that lead to cellular damage.

Mitochondrial Hypothesis: These small powerhouses of the cell are essential for energy generation. Mitochondrial function may deteriorate as we age, resulting in lower energy production and perhaps contributing to age-related disorders. Exercise, which stimulates and trains your mitochondria, might help them become more efficient, thus halting the decrease.

Theory of Telomeres: Telomeres, like the plastic tips on shoelaces, are protective caps at the ends of chromosomes. These telomeres shorten with each cell division, ultimately reaching a critical point where the cell can no longer function correctly. Certain dietary choices, such as ingesting omega-3 fatty acids found in fish, have been shown in studies to help preserve telomere length and improve cellular health.

Theory of Epigenetics: Consider DNA to be noted on a musical score, and epigenetics to be the conductor who determines which notes are performed loudly and which are soft. Environmental variables such as nutrition, stress, and exercise may all have an impact on epigenetic changes, altering the volume of specific genes' expression. This fascinating area brings up the possibility of modifying aging processes by "reprogramming" gene expression via lifestyle choices.

Lifestyle Decisions as a Conductor:

Diet: What you consume genuinely nurtures your cell symphony. A diet high in fruits, vegetables, and whole grains contains vitamins, minerals, and antioxidants that protect against cellular damage and inflammation. Excess sugar, processed meals, and unhealthy fats, on the other hand, may contribute to age-related disorders and hasten the aging process.

Exercise: Consider exercise to be a workout for your mitochondria, increasing their efficiency and encouraging energy generation. Even brisk walking may improve cardiovascular health, build muscles and bones, and even boost cognitive function. It's never too late to start moving and receive the advantages as you age.

Stress Reduction: Chronic stress disrupts the rhythm and melody of your symphony by acting like a discordant note. Meditation, yoga, and mindfulness techniques may help manage stress hormones and restore peace to your cells, building a more robust and adaptive internal environment.

Sleep:Your brain and body both heal and maintain themselves when you sleep. Prioritizing excellent sleep permits your cells to replenish and fight off free radicals and inflammation. To keep your internal symphony humming properly, aim for 7-8 hours of peaceful sleep each night.

Exceptional Aging Case Studies:

Jeanne Calment: The French lady who holds the record for the longest human lifetime (122 years!) credits her longevity to a good diet, modest exercise, and a happy attitude toward life. Interestingly, she also drank a glass of port wine every day, indicating that balance, rather than full abstention, may be important for certain aspects.

Dharma Singh Khalsa, Dr. This 87-year-old yoga teacher maintains incredible strength and flexibility, owing to diligent yoga practice, a vegetarian diet, and a profound connection to his faith. His narrative demonstrates the enormous potential for mind-body connection in healthy aging.

Emily Morano: An Italian supercentenarian who lived to the age of 117 attributed her long life to a simple diet of coffee, spaghetti, and eggs, as well as not worrying about things she couldn't control. This instance emphasizes the significance of individual variation and implies that there is no one-size-fits-all strategy for unusual aging.

These are only a few instances; there are innumerable inspirational tales of people who have matured gracefully and conquered obstacles.

2

Chapter 2: The Changing Body: From Cell Renewal to Physical Transformations

Our bodies are a magnificent tapestry constructed from billions of cells that are continually renewing and changing. Time, on the other hand, makes its imprint on this tapestry, adding changes that may be baffling, irritating, and even scary at times. However, the path of bodily metamorphosis in aging is not one of inevitability.

Goodbye, Cellular Innocence: Cells divide with young zeal in our youth, reproducing and regenerating with apparently infinite vitality. However, as we become older, this process slows down. Telomeres, or the protective caps on chromosomes, shrink with each cycle, ultimately leading to cellular retirement. This, however, does not portend disaster. Understanding the science of cellular aging enables us to help this process by making healthy lifestyle choices. A diet high in antioxidants and phytochemicals found in fruits and vegetables may help protect cells from aging. Even light exercise stimulates cellular regeneration and increases the effectiveness of our internal powerhouses, the mitochondria.

Metamorphosis of Muscles: Youthful muscles may seem to lose their bounce as they age. Muscle mass normally diminishes, resulting in reduced strength and an increased risk of injury. This, however, is not a one-way street! Resistance training, even with low weights or bodyweight exercises, may reverse muscle deterioration. It's not only about vanity when it comes to building and maintaining muscle mass; it's also about retaining independence, reducing falls, and increasing metabolism. Lift those weights and watch your body dance to a new beat of strength.

Bones in a Juggling Act: As we age, our bones, which were once strong pillars, may become thinner and more prone to shatter. Osteoporosis, known as the "silent thief of bone density," is a serious hazard, especially to women. But don't fret! The powerful duo of bone health, calcium, and vitamin D, may aid in the rebuilding and strengthening of your internal framework. A diet high in essential nutrients, supplemented as needed, along with weight-bearing sports such as dancing or walking, may keep your bones dancing the tango of resilience.

The Symphony of the Senses: Sight, hearing, taste, smell, and touch are all portals to the universe, and their melodies may vary as we mature. Presbyopia, or the progressive loss of close vision, may demand the use of reading glasses, but it does not have to dampen your enthusiasm for books. Hearing aids may intensify life's whispers, and even the sense of smell, with its strange link to memory, can be nourished via olfactory stimulation. Celebrate your sensory orchestra's unique symphony, accept the modifications, and explore new ways to perceive the world via your ever-evolving sensory orchestra.

A Mind on the Move: Memory may become hazy, and recall of knowledge may not be as quick as it once was. However, cognitive decline is not unavoidable. The Mozart of brain health, and mental stimulation, can keep your neurons blazing and synapses dancing. Learn a new language, solve difficult puzzles, and participate in social interactions—these are the batons that orchestrate the cognitive agility symphony. Keep in mind that periodic memory lapses are not always a sign of impending doom; they are just reminders that our brains are continuously reorganizing, forming new connections, and adapting to the shifting landscape of time.

Embrace Change: The evolving body is a teacher, a storyteller, and a witness to the great voyage of time. Learn its language, rhythms, and wisdom whispers. Celebrate the remaining power and tenacity, the new chapters that are emerging, and the unique symphony that your body now performs. We may negotiate the landscape of physical alteration with elegance, curiosity, and the persistent confidence that our bodies have the potential to surprise and inspire even amid time's dance.

Embracing the Kaleidoscope: Body Positivity and Aging Transformation

Aging and the changing body may be a bittersweet tango. While we may lament the loss of our young vigor, a powerful dose of body positivity may change this dance into a joyful waltz.

Rather than seeing wrinkles as war wounds, consider them to be maps of laughing, pleasure, and adventures inscribed on our skin. The aches and pains become whispers of the tales we carry in our bodies, testaments to marathons ran, mountains climbed, and lives thoroughly lived.

This adjustment in viewpoint is critical since our mental health and stress management have a direct influence on our physical health. Chronic stress is the unwanted conductor, destabilizing the symphony of hormones and immunological function. Relaxation activities such as meditation, yoga, and spending time in nature may help to balance the internal symphony, improving cellular repair and increasing our resistance to age-related decline.

It is critical to tailor exercise, diet, and cognitive stimulation to various age groups to maintain the body and mind healthy.

****For the Active Fortys and Fifties:** High-intensity interval training (HIIT) improves cardiovascular and metabolic health, while a Mediterranean diet rich in fruits, vegetables, and healthy fats fuels the body for further exploration.

Learning new abilities such as coding or calligraphy keep the neurons moving.

For Ladies in their Sixties and Seventies: Low-impact workouts such as swimming or yoga help to preserve agility and balance, while bone-supporting foods such as yogurt and leafy greens are essential. Puzzle evenings and lively discussions with loved ones keep the intellect fresh and social relationships alive.

For the Aged Eighties and Up: Gentle walks and chair yoga keep the body moving while eating gut-friendly foods and keeping hydrated promote internal wellbeing. Sharing life experiences and reminiscing with relatives keeps the mind busy and ties us to our beloved history.

3

Chapter 3: Mind Matters: Developing a Vibrant Inner Landscape in Later Life

As we travel through life, the mind, that amazing maze of ideas, memories, and emotions, experiences interesting modifications. While concerns about cognitive decline may loom big in the aging narrative, let's change the focus to a more powerful viewpoint. This chapter isn't about clinging to the hard grasp of youth; it's about nurturing a lively inner landscape in which cerebral agility, emotional well-being, and a sense of purpose dance in unison.

Debunking a Myth: Memory Loss and Mental Decline

The dreaded memory lapse - when the perfect word slips away, leaving you stumbling in a fog. But, before you leap to conclusions, keep in mind that forgetfulness is not the same as dementia or cognitive deterioration. Like well-traveled libraries, our brains continuously rearrange information, cutting certain paths and reinforcing others. While this process might be unpleasant at times, it is a sign of a dynamic, adaptive mind.

The Neuron Symphony: Keeping the Music Playing

Consider your brain to be a busy symphony, with neurons acting as instruments and synapses as the numerous connections between them. The task then becomes maintaining this symphony in tune. Intellectual stimulation, known as the Mozart of mental health, is essential. Learning a new language, solving difficult puzzles, or just participating in interesting discussions may build neural connections and increase cognitive reserve, the brain's buffer against age-related deterioration.

Fueling the Mental Engine: Mind-Body Nutrition

To work efficiently, the brain, like any high-performance engine, requires the proper fuel. A diet high in omega-3 fatty acids, which are found in fish and flaxseeds, antioxidants from fruits and vegetables, and B vitamins help fuel your neurons and protect you against cognitive loss. Don't underestimate the need for drinking; dehydration may cause slow thinking and memory lapses. So, keep your brain engine humming with a bright, healthy fuel tank.

Embracing the Spectrum in Later Years: The Dance of Emotions

Aging is a period of emotional transformation as well as physical changes. Loss, loss, and changes may bring on a slew of emotions, leaving us feeling vulnerable and adrift. But keep in mind that these emotions are not unwanted visitors; they are messengers conveying precious messages. We may traverse this emotional terrain with grace and resilience if we acknowledge and process our feelings with self-compassion and acceptance.

Mindfulness and Meditation for Inner Peace

Mindfulness and meditation emerge as powerful techniques for inner serenity amid racing thoughts and anxiety. Stepping back to watch your thoughts without judgment, for example, trains the mind to be present in the moment, lowering stress and boosting emotional well-being. Consider your mind to be a tumultuous ocean; mindfulness and meditation are the anchors that help you traverse the waves with more peace and clarity.

Social Connections: The Belonging Symphon

Humans are social beings that are hardwired for connection. Isolation and loneliness, on the other hand, may pose considerable dangers to mental health in later life. Nurturing meaningful connections with friends, family, and loved ones is more than simply a source of happiness; it is also a cornerstone of emotional wellness. Sharing our humor, stories, and experiences increases our feeling of belonging and serves as an essential support network during difficult times.

Finding Purpose: A Compass for a Meaningful Life

Even in our latter years, a feeling of purpose, that guiding light that provides meaning to our lives, is essential. Finding activities that light your flame and contribute to something more than yourself, whether it's giving your time, following artistic pursuits, or just spending quality time with loved ones, may provide enormous pleasure and fulfillment. Remember that purpose is a voyage of constant investigation and discovery, not a predetermined goal.

Embrace the Journey, Celebrate the Change

Aging does not guarantee cognitive decline and emotional misery. We may build a lively inner landscape where mental agility, emotional well-being, and a sense of purpose grow by stimulating our brains with academic stimulation, proper diet, and emotional awareness. Accept the inevitable changes, enjoy the knowledge and resilience that come with age, and realize that your mind, like a well-tended garden, may continue to flourish with beauty and wonder throughout your life.

personal anecdotes or case studies of individuals who have maintained cognitive function and emotional well-being in later years.

The Puzzle Queen, Grandma Evelyn: Evelyn, 85, has the laser concentration of a hawk when it comes to crossword puzzles, her head bursting with wordplay and information. Her mystery? A lifelong love of study, a daily crossword puzzle habit, and a thriving social network keep her intellect on its toes. Her experience reminds us that academic stimulation may keep the mind sharp and the soul engaged.

***The Dancing Spirit, Uncle Leo:** Leo may have withdrawn into dread and seclusion after being diagnosed with Parkinson's disease in his sixties. But he chose happiness instead. He welcomed Zumba lessons, where he found friendship and rhythm. He's the star of the senior center dance floor now, at 78, his laughter resounding through the corridors, an encouragement to everyone who sees his passion soar. Leo's tale demonstrates the importance of social interaction and finding pleasure in exercise, even in the face of adversity.

Community Gardener Ms. Rodriguez: Ms. Rodriguez, 92, nurtures a communal garden with the zeal of a teenager. She finds purpose and connection when kneeling in the dirt, her hands nurturing seedlings. Her vibrant garden reflects the vigor inside her. Ms. Rodriguez's narrative emphasizes the significance of purpose and giving back, reminding us that age is no barrier to making a difference in the world.

The Lullaby of Sleep and Its Importance in Brain Health

Sleep is like our brains' nightly orchestra conductor, directing a symphony of crucial activities that keep our minds sharp and cognitive function on the pitch. Strange things happen when we drift away:

Memory organization: Our brains replay, consolidate, and arrange memories from the day, ensuring that they are retained for future use. Consider it like putting essential papers aside for later use.

Toxins removed: Sleep, like a good cleaner, cleans up the waste products that accumulate in our brains during the day, avoiding mental clutter overload.

Recharge your brainpower: Your brain, like your phone, needs charging. Sleep recharges your brain batteries, increasing your alertness, attention, and problem-solving abilities the following day.

Emotional control: A good night's sleep also aids in the regulation of our emotions. We are more prone to irritation, anxiety, and mood changes when we are sleep-deprived. As a result, sleep acts as a salve for our mental well-being.

Consider sleep to be a necessary investment in your brain's health and cognitive performance, rather than a luxury. Chronic sleep deprivation has been linked to memory issues, trouble focusing, and an increased risk of dementia, according to research.

Here are some suggestions to keep your brain's conductor humming the pleasant sleep lullaby:

Establish a consistent sleep schedule: Go to bed and get up at the same time every day, including on weekends, to train your body's internal clock.

Create a peaceful bedtime routine: Relax before bed by taking a warm bath, reading a book, or listening to quiet music.

Make your bedroom sleep-friendly: Keep it dark, quiet, and cool for at least an hour before going to bed. Invest in blackout curtains, earplugs, and a comfy mattress.

Addressing sleep disorders: If you have persistent sleep issues such as insomnia or sleep apnea, see a doctor. Treatment may enhance sleep quality and general health dramatically.

Get regular exercise: However, avoid hard activities too close to sleep. These might cause sleep disruption, so consume them in moderation earlier in the day.

Nap power: Short, well-timed naps may improve alertness and cognitive performance, especially in older persons.

You can guarantee your brain's orchestra conductor maintains the music of clarity, memory, and well-being playing wonderfully every night by prioritizing sleep and adopting good sleep practices. Remember that a good night's sleep is a gift you give your brain, and it will repay you with a symphony of cognitive ability for years to come.

Cultivating a Vibrant Mind: Tools and Advice for Later Life

practical methods and resources to foster cognitive agility, emotional well-being, and resilience in later years. some concrete actions people may take to keep their wits bright, spirits high, and relationships strong.

Stimulation of Cognitive Function:

Brain Training Games: Apps such as Lumosity and Elevate provide a fun and easy approach to improving memory, concentration, and problem-solving abilities.

Learn a New Language: Keeping your brain flexible and adaptive by learning a new language opens access to new cultures and relationships.

Reading and Puzzles: Reading promotes critical thinking and inventiveness, and puzzles such as crossword puzzles and sudoku improve memory and mental agility.

Creative Activities: Writing, drawing, music, or any creative effort keeps the mind agile and delves into previously untapped stores of creativity.

Social Engagement: Engaging in engaging discussions, attending lectures or seminars, and participating in group activities stimulates the mind while also fostering social bonds.

Mindfulness and Stress Reduction:

Meditation Apps like Headspace and Calm provide guided meditations for both beginners and seasoned practitioners, assisting in the cultivation of inner peace and stress reduction.

Yoga and Tai Chi: These mind-body activities promote relaxation and emotional well-being by combining gentle movement with breathwork and awareness.

Deep Breathing Exercises: Taking slow, deep breaths throughout the day may help to relax the nervous system and relieve tension.

Spending Time in Nature: Spending time in nature has been shown to improve cognitive performance and mood, as well as generate a feeling of serenity and connection.

Journaling: Writing down ideas and feelings may aid in the processing of tough emotions, tracking progress, and increasing self-awareness, all of which contribute to emotional well-being.

Overcoming Mental Health Obstacles:

Early Detection: Understanding the signs and symptoms of common mental health conditions such as depression and anxiety in later years is critical for prompt intervention.

Seeking Professional Help: If you are experiencing emotional difficulties, don't be afraid to seek professional help from a therapist or counselor. Early intervention may increase well-being and quality of life greatly.

Support Groups: Connecting with people going through similar experiences via support groups may give important understanding, empathy, and practical help.

Online services: Websites such as MentalHealth.gov and the National Alliance on Mental Illness (NAMI) provide information, support services, and tools to help people dealing with mental health issues.

Self-Care and Good Habits: Prioritizing sleep, good diet, and regular exercise contribute to general well-being and give a solid basis for dealing with mental health issues.

Technology as a Gateway, Not a Barrier:

Technology, which is sometimes seen as a barrier to aging, maybe a tremendous instrument for cognitive stimulation, social interaction, and resource access. Consider the following options:

Virtual Reality (VR) experiences: From visiting museums to playing memory games, VR can deliver brain-stimulating locations and activities.

Telehealth and online therapy: Online platforms make it easy to connect with mental health specialists and support groups, reducing geographic obstacles to treatment.

Social media and online communities: Using social media to communicate with friends and family, joining online groups based on interests, and engaging in forums may help prevent social isolation and establish meaningful relationships.

Learning applications and online courses: Technology facilitates lifelong learning by enabling people to explore new interests and keep their brains engaged at any age.

Digital storytelling and creative platforms: Sharing tales, images, and creative endeavors online may help people connect with loved ones while also instilling a feeling of purpose and participation.

4

Chapter 4: The Magic of Intergenerational Connections: Bridging the Generation Gap

L et us enter the dynamic realm of intergenerational relationships! This is about creating a tapestry of knowledge, fun, and mutual progress amongst generations, not merely filling social calendars.

Beyond Stereotypes: The Power of Relationship

Age is sometimes portrayed as a dividing line in the media, portraying an image of disconnected generations with nothing in common. However, the truth is considerably more lovely. Intergenerational interactions bridge the generational divide, forging bonds that benefit both the young and the elderly.

To the Next Generation:

* **Mentorship and Guidance:** As mentors and role models, older folks provide a wealth of insight and experience. They can help you navigate life's problems, create a profession, and learn vital life skills.

* **Historical Connection:** Grandparents and elders serve as living bridges to the past, providing anecdotes and personal descriptions of historical events and helping to shape a more complete grasp of history and culture.

* **Compassion and Perspective:** Interacting with older folks increases empathy and knowledge of the issues of aging. Young people grow in their sense of community and learn to appreciate the contributions of all generations.

Note To The Elderly:

* **Overcoming Loneliness:** Connecting with younger people promotes friendship while combating emotions of isolation. Grandchildren and younger friends provide joy, new energy, and a feeling of purpose.

* **Stimulation of Cognitive Function:** Keeping older minds alive and bright requires interaction with younger ones. Playing games, learning new technology, and exchanging tales all excite the mind and keep it nimble.

* **Remaining Connected to the Present:** Younger generations serve as ambassadors to the present, bringing older folks up to date on current trends, pop culture, and technical advances. This connection alleviates feelings of isolation and develops a sense of belonging.

Creating Meaningful Connections

Making intergenerational relationships isn't magic; it's deliberate action! Here are several ideas for igniting the flame:

* **Volunteer Together:** Find a subject that both of you are passionate about and volunteer together. Working together develops ties and promotes a feeling of common purpose.

* **Intergenerational Activities:** Host game evenings, culinary courses, or storytelling sessions to bring together people of various ages. Sharing shared interests and activities fosters discussion and laughter.

* **Technology Bridge:** Assist elderly folks in learning new technologies and connecting online with younger family members. Video conversations, social media sites, and game consoles may help families stay connected over long distances.

* **Storytelling Nights:** Invite grandparents and other seniors to share their life tales. These priceless testimonies give historical context, stir debate, and leave a legacy that links generations.

Remember that intergenerational relationships are about more than merely filling social calendars; they are about making genuine connections that benefit both sides' lives. Weaving a tapestry of empathy, understanding, and mutual development by developing these relationships, age is really only a number and that the human spirit, like an eternal flame, can transcend any distance and light the road towards a more connected and joyous world.

Let's alter the story of aging. Let us celebrate the power of intergenerational relationships and create a society where knowledge from the past dances with the vitality of the present, producing a symphony of belonging and shared delight.

Technology: Bridging Gaps and Nurturing Relationships in Later Years

we looked at the magic of social interaction and the profound bonds it creates in our lives, particularly as we become older. But, let's face it, distance, movement, and even shyness may make it difficult to cultivate these crucial ties. This is where technology comes in, not as a barrier, but as a bridge - a tremendous instrument for connecting and overcoming barriers.

Redefining Distance: Crossing Miles

Physical distance no longer equals separation. Technology such as video calls and messaging applications enable us to communicate face-to-face with loved ones anywhere in the globe in real-time. Through the magic of screens, a grandchild in another city may enjoy bedtime tales, celebrate milestones, and experience the warmth of their grandparent's presence. Families may meet virtually for virtual meals, exchange jokes and laughs, and keep connected despite physical distance.

Social Media: A Community and Discovery Platform

Social media platforms, which are frequently regarded with suspicion, may be effective instruments for establishing and sustaining social ties in later life. Online communities devoted to certain hobbies allow people to connect with others who have similar interests, exchange experiences, and find support. There is a virtual community for everyone, from gardening lovers to birdwatchers, history buffs to IT geeks, delivering a feeling of connection and shared hobbies.

Using Technology to Learn and Engage

Technology not only connects individuals, but it also offers doors to new experiences and learning possibilities. Individuals may acquire new skills, investigate novel subjects, and keep their brains busy by taking online courses, webinars, and interactive tutorials. A world of information and interaction is only a click away, from mastering video production to brushing up on a new language.

Digital Age Mindfulness and Wellbeing

While technology has many advantages, it is important to utilize it responsibly and mindfully. Setting screen time limits, emphasizing face-to-face conversations, and participating in offline activities are all vital for striking a good balance. To get the most advantages from technology, it must be used as a tool for connection rather than as a substitute for face-to-face conversations.

Reducing Isolation and Promoting Inclusion

Technology may be a lifesaver for those who have limited mobility or are isolated. Online therapy sessions make mental health help more accessible, while virtual support groups give a secure area to interact with others experiencing similar issues. Individuals may use technology to break away from isolation and create a network of support and understanding.

Keep in mind that technology is not a miracle answer; it is a tool that must be utilized with purpose and understanding. Individuals in their senior years may transcend geographical constraints, develop meaningful connections, and improve their lives with pleasure and purpose by utilizing their capacity for connection, learning, and community.

Let's reinvent the aging and technology story. Let us celebrate the power of digital connectivity and highlight how technology may enable people to live full, dynamic lives, connect with the world around them, and overcome age and distance barriers. We can work together to build a world where technology bridges rather than increases barriers and nurtures a symphony of connectivity across generations and geographical borders.

5

Chapter 5: Financial Planning for Older Age Security and Independence

As we go through life, the environment changes, as do our financial demands and objectives. Planning for the future, which was previously a distant horizon, has become a more immediate and practical reality. This is when financial foresight comes into play, as a lighthouse directing us to stability and independence in our elderly years.

Beyond the Myths: Rethinking Financial Planning for Seniors

In later years, fear and uncertainty can distort the debate about financial planning. Myths about scarcity and decline build an image of retirement as a financial cliff edge. However, this is far from the reality! Financial foresight is about making educated decisions and taking charge of your financial future, allowing you to keep your preferred lifestyle and independence.

The Importance of Early Planning: A Seed Planted Today Will Bloom Tomorrow

The golden rule of financial planning is to begin early. Small measures made now, like planting a seed that develops into a robust and powerful tree, may bloom into a secure and satisfying future. Whether you're in your forties, fifties, or beyond, the sooner you start, the more time you have to lay a firm financial foundation.

- Building Your Financial Fortress: Essential Stability Pillars Consider your financial future to be a gorgeous castle that is both sturdy and durable. Here are the fundamental pillars upon which it will be built:
- Retirement Savings: It is important to contribute to your retirement accounts, such as IRAs and 401(k)s, regularly. To enhance your savings plan, take advantage of workplace matching programs and consider getting expert advice.
- Debt Management:Address current debt. Prioritize high-interest debts and devise a repayment strategy to free up future income for other requirements.
- Diversification of Income: Do not depend only on retirement income. Consider generating extra income sources to complement your pension and social security, such as freelance work, rental properties, or even part-time employment.
- Estate Planning: Make plans for the future by drafting a will and a power of attorney. This guarantees that your assets are allocated how you intend and protects your loved ones in the event of incapacity.
- Review and Modify: Your budget is not a static document. Review your progress regularly, alter your plans as appropriate, and adapt to changing conditions.

More Than Numbers: The Human Aspects of Financial Planning

Financial planning is much more than just spreadsheets and figures; it is about your life, your desires, and your goals. *Consider the following considerations while developing your strategy:*

- Lifestyle Objectives: What type of retirement lifestyle do you envision? Do you want to explore the globe, pursue hobbies, or spend time with family and friends? Define your objectives and adjust your financial strategy appropriately.

- Healthcare Needs: Healthcare expenditures might climb as we age. Consider prospective medical bills and choices such as long-term care insurance or supplementary health plans.
- Family and Legacies: Planning for the future of your family is an essential component of financial foresight. Consider how you would provide for and ensure the well-being of your loved ones when you are gone.

Tools and Resources for Your Financial Journey:

Navigating the financial world may seem difficult, but there are various resources and tools available to assist you along the way:

- Financial Advisors: Seek professional advice from a qualified financial advisor who can tailor a plan to your specific needs and risk tolerance.
- Online Tools and Calculators: Use online resources such as budgeting apps, retirement calculators, and debt management tools to gain insights and track your progress.

Keep in mind that financial foresight is a journey, not a destination. It is about being proactive, seeking assistance when necessary, and changing your strategy as life unfolds. With a constructive attitude toward financial planning, you may create a secure and rewarding future, assuring independence and peace of mind in your elderly years.

Defying the Odds: Stories of Resilience and Triumph in the Face of Financial Difficulties

We discussed the significance of financial planning for a secure and independent future. However, reality seldom follows flawless plans, and financial difficulties may develop even for the most thorough planners. Resilience, resourcefulness, and a good attitude come into play here, weaving fascinating tales of older persons who defy expectations and flourish despite limited resources.

Introducing Agnes, the Frugal Foodie: Agnes, 72, lives alone in a little apartment. She was widowed young and faced years of raising her children on a small budget. Nonetheless, her little kitchen buzzes with activity, filled with the smells of delectable food. Agnes is a master of frugal cooking, preparing healthy and delectable meals using coupons, local grocery stores, and inventive recipes. Her apartment is filled with laughter and the pleasure of family connection as she holds monthly potlucks for her grandkids. Agnes' enthusiasm isn't dimmed by financial constraints; she takes satisfaction in simple pleasures like watching sunsets from her balcony, tending to her rooftop garden, and helping at a community center.

Michael, the Tech-Savvy Senior: Michael faced early retirement and a limited income after being diagnosed with a chronic ailment in his late 50s. Undaunted, he accepted technology as his lifeline. He learned to code online, started a freelance web design company from home, and now assists other seniors in navigating the digital world. His earnings enhance his pension, and his technological abilities keep him cognitively bright and linked to a worldwide society. Michael's narrative demonstrates that age does not impede learning and reinvention; even financial difficulties may serve as springboards for development and unexpected success.

The Community Architect, Eleanor: Eleanor, at the age of 85, is a live example of the importance of giving back. She refused to be alone despite living in a remote location with little support for elderly folks. She mobilized her neighbors, arranged fundraising events, and obtained funds to construct a senior community center. Today, the facility is alive with activity, providing meals, fitness courses, and social gatherings. Eleanor's tale demonstrates how collective initiative and community spirit may overcome financial constraints. Her proactive attitude not only enhanced her own life but also the lives of many others.

These are just a few snippets from the tapestry of resilience created by older adults. Each narrative defies preconceptions and demonstrates the human spirit's incredible capacity to adapt, invent, and find pleasure in the face of adversity.

Calming the Storm: Addressing Common Concerns and Anxieties About Long-Term Financial Planning

This chapter has traversed the terrain of financial foresight, emphasizing its relevance in achieving independence and peace of mind. However, the very thought of preparing for an unknown future may cause anxiety and concern. Let's address some of the most prevalent worries that cloud our judgment and give real methods to quiet the financial storm inside.

The Fear of the Unknown:

The future, particularly in financial terms, might seem to be vast and undiscovered land. Because of the uncertainty, it is impossible to foresee a safe future.

- Reassurance: Keep in mind that you are not alone on this path. Millions of people face identical concerns. Concentrate on what you can manage, such as your current activities and proactive planning. Accept uncertainty as a chance to explore, adapt, and gain resilience.

- Problem with Starting Late: A typical complaint is, "I should have started earlier!" While an early start is preferable, even a late start is beneficial. Every step, no matter how tiny, gets you closer to your objectives. Don't waste time lamenting the past; instead, grab the present and construct a secure future one step at a time.
- Solution: Seek expert advice from a financial adviser who can create a strategy based on your present circumstances and remaining years. Estimate retirement requirements and monitor progress using online tools and services. Begin with tiny, attainable savings objectives and gradually build momentum.

Burden of Debt:

Existing debt might seem like a stumbling block, pulling you down and impeding your financial development.

- Reassurance: Remember that debt management is an option. Prioritize high-interest debts, investigate consolidation opportunities, and establish a realistic repayment strategy. Don't allow debt to control your life; you can conquer it.
- Solution: Create a detailed debt management strategy that includes payments, deadlines, and prospective revenue sources. Seek the help of debt counselors or financial consultants. Celebrate each debt-reduction milestone to keep your spirits up along the road.

Costs of Healthcare:

The worry of increased healthcare expenditures in the future is a significant source of anxiety.

- Reassurance: While life is unpredictable, cautious preparation may help to reduce stress. Investigate and get acquainted with various healthcare alternatives, such as Medicare and supplementary insurance programs. Consider long-term care choices and talk them over with your family.
- Solution: Investigate government subsidies and programs for the elderly.

Contribute to Health Savings Accounts (HSAs) to offset future medical costs. Maintain a healthy lifestyle to reduce prospective healthcare expenditures and emphasize preventative care.

I'm Overwhelmed:

Financial planning's sheer complexity may be intimidating, leading to delay and inactivity.

- Reassurance: Financial planning should be broken down into achievable segments. Concentrate on one thing at a time, such as budgeting, debt management, or retirement savings. Don't be scared to seek expert assistance; it may relieve stress and bring comfort.
- Solution: To simplify hard processes, use existing resources such as internet tools, calculators, and budgeting applications. Begin small, praise your accomplishments, and gradually increase your confidence in your financial knowledge and abilities. Keep in mind that even tiny actions contribute to considerable improvement over time.

In later years, financial planning isn't about eliminating anxieties; it's about arming ourselves with knowledge, resources, and a positive mindset to navigate them effectively. By addressing common concerns and offering practical solutions, we can empower individuals to embrace control, prioritize action, and build a secure and fulfilling future, regardless of the financial storms they may face.

Keep in mind that you are not alone on this path. Let us go on this journey together, equipped with knowledge, resilience, and a firm conviction in our potential to create a bright and happy future one step at a time.

6

Chapter 6: Nourishing Your Body: A Recipe Book for Healthy Eating

Our bodies, like faithful friends, accompany us through the chapters of life. And, just as a loyal horse needs good nutrition to carry us far, our temple of flesh and bone craves delectable and nutritious feed to flourish in later years. In this chapter, we'll go on a gastronomic excursion, busting misconceptions and discovering the exquisite joys of healthy eating at a later age.

Beyond Restrictive Regimes: Reframing the Aging and Food Narrative

Aging, which is sometimes depicted as a time of nutritional limitations and boring meals, deserves a gastronomic revolution! Forget about the boring chicken and boiled veggies of old clichés. In later life, nourishing your body means enjoying a diverse tapestry of tastes, textures, and cultural influences, all while prioritizing health and well-being. It's about realizing that becoming older isn't a barrier to culinary delight, but rather a doorway to a new chapter of delicious and healthful inquiry.

The Taste Symphony: Balancing Deliciousness and Nutritional Needs

Consider your plate to be a musical score, with each element serving as a harmonizing note in a symphony of flavor and well-being. *Here are some crucial chords to play for a nutritious and tasty melody:*

- Fruits & Vegetables: These brilliant hues are rich in antioxidants and vitamins, benefiting your health while also pleasing your palette. find new types, experiment with colorful salads, and find the roasted veggies' secret delicacy.
- Whole Grains: These complex carbs provide prolonged energy, similar to a slow and steady drumming throughout the day. Replace white bread with whole-wheat alternatives, quinoa and brown rice, and whole-grain cereals for their nutty deliciousness.
- Light Protein: These important building elements, whether fish, chicken, or beans, keep your muscles healthy and your body satisfied. Grill, bake or poach for light and tasty alternatives, and for extra diversity, look into vegetarian sources like lentils and tofu.
- Fitness Fats: Don't be afraid of fat! Choose the healthy type, which can be found in avocados, almonds, and olive oil and helps to lubricate your joints, protect your heart, and give flavor to your meals. Drizzle olive oil over your salad, chew on nuts, and enjoy the creamy richness of avocado toast (in moderation, of course!).

The Influence of Home Cooking: Your Kitchen as a Canvas

Put an end to manufactured foods and take charge of your culinary canvas! Home cooking allows you to choose fresh ingredients, regulate portion proportions, and experiment with tastes to suit your preferences. It's a kind of self-care, a creative release, and a fun opportunity to reconnect with loved ones over meals.

- Spice Up Your Life: Herbs and spices are more than simply taste enhancers; they're also powerful health friends. Turmeric's anti-inflammatory capabilities, ginger's digestive advantages, and rosemary's memory-boosting potential – weave these culinary threads into your recipes for a symphony of flavor and well-being.

· Hydration Harmony: Water conducts the symphony, keeping your body's orchestra in tune. To add a pleasant touch to your water, infuse it with fruits, herbs, or even cucumbers, and avoid sugary beverages.

· Mindful Munching: Pay attention to your body's signals. Enjoy each mouthful, avoid distractions while eating, and quit when you're satisfied. Mindful eating promotes a positive connection with food and helps to avoid overeating.

Overcoming Obstacles: Myths Busted and Solutions Provided

The route to delightful and healthful eating in older years is not without challenges. Let's tackle some frequent obstacles to ensure a comfortable gastronomic ride:

Myth: **"Cooking for one is boring and impractical."**

Solution:Accept leftovers! Cook in bigger amounts and freeze parts for later use. Investigate mini-recipes designed for single servings, and invest in multi-purpose kitchen gadgets that make cooking for one enjoyable and efficient.

***Problem: "Loss of taste and smell makes food bland."**

Solution: Experiment with different textures and tastes. Try different culinary techniques like grilling or roasting, and experiment with colorful veggies with diverse flavors. Share meals with loved ones to increase the social component and pleasure of dining.

Disappointment: "Eating healthy is expensive."

Solution: To efficiently budget, plan your meals, take advantage of grocery store promotions, and learn to cook from scratch. Choose low-cost protein sources like beans and lentils, produce your herbs, and look for healthy substitutes for pricey goods.

Remember that sustaining your body in later years is about enjoying the joy of food, the pleasure of cooking, and the power of taste to energize your body and spirit.You may create a culinary experience by adopting a balanced approach, stressing fresh ingredients, and experimenting with tastes.

7

Chapter 7: Move Your Way to Health: Exercise Techniques for People of All Fitness Levels and Ages

The human body thrives on movement, much like a well-oiled machine. However, as life unfolds, the speed varies, and the once-familiar rhythm of exercise requires delicate rescoring. Not to worry, because in this chapter, we celebrate the delight of "moving your way to health," creating a workout symphony for every fitness level and age, demonstrating that age is only a number when it comes to the lively music of a healthy life.

More Than a Treadmill: Redefining Exercise in Later Life

Forget the tired stereotypes of elderly aerobics and dusty treadmills. Later-life exercise is a bright tapestry woven with varied motions, specific objectives, and the simple delight of rediscovering your body's possibilities. It's not about pushing boundaries or chasing gym bunnies; it's about appreciating your own body's particular rhythm and discovering activities that spark your soul and nurture your well-being.

The Harmony of Movement: Discovering Your Ideal Tempo

Your workout program should reflect the diversity of your body's requirements and aspirations, much as a musical group finds its rhythm with a range of instruments. ***Here are some harmonic tones to use in your movement symphony:***

- Cardio Cadence: Gently stroll, swim, or dance to your favorite sounds to keep your heart singing. Discover activities that you love, pay attention to your body's speed, and gradually increase intensity as you feel comfortable.
- Strength Serenade: Use modest resistance training with bands, weights, or even your bodyweight to build your muscle choir. Squats, lunges, and light weightlifting may help you maintain your balance, avoid falls, and keep your bones healthy.
- Flexibility Finesse: Use stretches, yoga positions, or tai chi moves to keep your body fluid. These delicate movements help to keep your joints flexible, enhance your posture, and produce a feeling of serenity and concentration.
- Balancing Ballet: Incorporate balancing exercises into your regimen to glide through life with confidence. Walking on your toes, standing on one leg, and tai chi may help you avoid falls and keep your motions steady.

The Joy of Movement: Rediscovering the Power of Play

Remember how much fun you used to have playing games as a kid? Reconnect with your fun side! Infuse your routine with activities that inspire laughter and fire your inner kid, whether it's a brisk trek in nature, a lively game of badminton with pals, or enrolling in a dancing class. Movement is about reconnecting with the simple joy of being alive, not only about bodily rewards.

Overcoming Obstacles: Aligning with Your Body's Needs

The melodies of life may occasionally become minor chords, revealing physical limits or health worries. Even yet, the song of movement continues. ***Here's how you maintain the rhythm:***

- Listen to Your Body: Pain is not a conductor you should listen to. Modify workouts, take pauses as required, and put comfort ahead of pushing limitations. If the discomfort continues or you have any concerns, get medical attention.
- Improve and Adapt: Don't let constraints restrict your mobility. For people with physical limitations, chair exercises, water workouts, or even light yoga movements may be effective alternatives. Creativity and flexibility are essential for keeping the music going.
- Discover Your Tribe: Join a senior fitness class, locate a walking club, or find an exercise partner. Social engagement and shared purpose may liven up your routine and make physical activity more fun.

Keep in mind that exercising in later life is not about competing or reaching superhuman feats. It's about honoring your body's unique symphony, discovering things that make you happy, and nourishing your well-being with the soothing rhythm of movement. So tie up your shoes, put on your dance shoes, or just go for a stroll outdoors. Allow your body's music to take center stage as you dance your way to a healthier, happier self.

Moving the Melody: Simple Routines & Tips for Everyone

let's get down to business, creating individualized regimens for varied fitness levels and limits. Remember that the goal is to discover activities that you like and that are in sync with your body's natural rhythm.

For the Beginner's Beat:

- Begin slowly and gently with brief walks, mild stretches, or chair exercises. Pay attention to your body and gradually increase the time and intensity as you get more comfortable.

- Embrace Everyday Movement: Move a part of your everyday routine. Take the stairs instead of the elevator, park farther away, and enjoy your housework. Every step is important!
- Determine the Fun Factor:Choose activities that you love, such as dancing to music, swimming in a warm pool, or taking a mild yoga session with friends. Movement should be enjoyable rather than arduous.

For the Consistent Stepper:

- Expand on the Fundamentals: Increase the time and intensity of your walks, include resistance bands into your routines, or attempt bodyweight exercises like squats and lunges.
- Explore Interval Training: To increase your fitness level and burn more calories, alternate between moderate and high-intensity exercises for brief bursts.
- Join a Group Fitness Class: Group sessions provide friendship, encouragement, and planned routines that are geared to different fitness levels. Consider low-impact dancing courses, water aerobics, or senior fitness programs.

For the Melodious Mover:

- Challenge Yourself: Push your boundaries safely by adding weights, increasing the difficulty of your workouts, or attempting new activities like hiking or cycling.
- Cross-Train for Variety: Vary your workouts to target various muscle groups and avoid boredom. Incorporate aerobic, weight training, balancing exercises, and flexibility stretches into your weekly schedule.
- Embrace Technology: Use fitness apps, online training videos, or wearable trackers to measure your progress, track steps, and get new exercise ideas.

For Those Who Have Restrictions:

- Adapt and Improvise: Change workouts to meet your specific requirements. Use chairs for balancing exercises, water workouts if joint discomfort prevents you from doing so on land, or light yoga positions for increased flexibility.
- Pay Attention to Your Body: Pain should never be in charge of your movement symphony. Take pauses as required, alter activities as needed, and seek medical attention if discomfort continues or you have any concerns.
- Find Helpful Resources: Contact physical therapists, adaptive fitness trainers, or senior fitness facilities that provide specific programs for people with disabilities.

Keep in mind that these are merely beginning points. Make your regimen fit your requirements and tastes, and don't be hesitant to try new things. ***Here are some more suggestions to keep the music playing***:

- Celebrate minor triumphs and set reasonable objectives.
- Find a workout partner for extra incentive and support.
- Spend money on comfy clothes and supportive shoes.
- Congratulate yourself for adhering to your schedule.
- Most importantly, enjoy yourself and the process.

It's not about attaining Olympian feats or pursuing gym bunnies in your older years. It's about developing your unique movement symphony that feeds your body, awakens your pleasure, and keeps you dancing to the lively beat of life. So, grab your movement instrument, choose your exact pace, and let the music lead you to a better, happier self.

Beyond Physical Gains: Embracing Movement's Mental and Emotional Symphony

we looked at the enticing melody of movement, creating individualized fitness programs for each individual. But exercise is more than simply shaping muscles or increasing stamina; it's like orchestrating a full-body symphony in which physical movement orchestrates a chorus of mental and emotional well-being. Let's dig into the symphony's secret notes, exposing the significant influence exercise may have on stress reduction, mood improvement, and cognitive clarity in later life.

How to Silence the Stressful Cymbals:

Life's difficulties may often seem like a cacophony of tension, leaving us tense and overwhelmed. However, exercise provides a relaxing contrast by serving as a natural stress reliever. Endorphins, nature's mood-elevating chemicals, are released by our bodies during physical exercise, helping to melt away concerns and generate a sensation of peace. Regular exercise may be your tranquilizer without the side effects, slowly reducing stress hormones and adjusting your mood to a more harmonic frequency, whether it's a brisk stroll in nature, a soothing yoga session, or a vigorous dancing class.

How to Tune the Moodful Bells:

Exercise has mental and emotional advantages that go beyond stress reduction. Regular physical exercise is a powerful antidepressant, increasing serotonin and dopamine levels in the brain, which are both important for mood regulation and treating depression. The clouds of negativity gradually lift as you move your body, to be replaced with a brighter view and a renewed feeling of hope. Exercise acts as a natural mood lifter, enabling you to tap into a reservoir of joy and inner serenity, allowing you to confront life's obstacles with a more resilient and cheerful attitude.

Improving Cognitive Chimes:

The music of movement resonates not only in the present but also in the future, enhancing cognitive function and safeguarding memory. Regular exercise has been proven in studies to increase attention, concentration, and cognitive flexibility, lowering the risk of dementia and Alzheimer's disease later in life. It's like getting a brain boost every day, keeping your mental gears greased and working smoothly, and helping you to negotiate life's challenges with clarity and confidence.

Remember, the mental and emotional benefits of exercise are not just temporary Over time, regular physical activity can:

- Improve your sleep quality, leaving you feeling refreshed and rejuvenated.
- Boost your self-esteem and confidence, allowing you to take on new tasks.
- Promote a feeling of belonging and community, particularly while engaging in group fitness programs.** * **Reduce the risk of chronic illnesses, therefore improving overall health**

Do not underestimate the potential of movement to promote mental and emotional well-being. Every walk, stretch, and dance motion becomes a note in the symphony of your life. So, grab your movement instrument, select your right pace, and let the music lead you to a healthier, happier, and more resilient self.

Here are some more techniques to boost exercise's mental and emotional benefits:

- While exercising, practice mindfulness by paying attention to your breath and body sensations.
- Select activities that you love, making moving a pleasure rather than a job.
- Exercise outside whenever possible to connect with nature and increase your mood.
- Connect with loved ones while exercising to encourage social contact and support.
- Celebrate your accomplishments, no matter how little, to remain inspired and keep the song flowing.

Let's reinvent the story of age and mobility. Let us rejoice in the full-body symphony that exercise creates, where physical benefits merge seamlessly with mental and emotional well-being. One joyous stride at a time, we can move a strong instrument for a bright and fulfilled future.

Keep in mind that the conductor's baton is inside you. Pick it up, accept the rhythm of movement, and let the music of your life emerge, vivid note after bright note.

8

Chapter 8: Rejuvenation and Rest: The Importance of Sleep for Wellbeing

Our bodies, like well-worn books, need moments of stop, pages to flip, and chapters to rest as we walk the chapters of life. And none of these calm regions is more important than the world of sleep. In this chapter, we'll dig into the enchanted realm of slumber, examining the critical role that great sleep plays in our well-being, especially as we become older.

Beyond the Sandman's Dust: Reframing the Sleep Narrative in Later Life

Forget the clichés of elderly people napping in rocking chairs. In later life, quality sleep isn't a luxury; it's a need, a rich tapestry woven with health advantages that go well beyond ordinary slumber. It's about recharging our thoughts and bodies' batteries and ready them for the experiences that the morning offers.

The Sleep Symphony: Understanding the Stages and Their Benefits

Consider sleep to be a musical composition, with each stage representing a harmonic flow. Let us investigate these movements and their critical roles:

• *NREM 1 & 2: These calm melodies help us transition from consciousness to sleep by decreasing our heart rate and relieving muscular tension.

- Deep Sleep: Like a deep cello solo, this restorative movement revitalizes our bodies, rebuilding tissues and increasing immunity.
- REM Sleep: This playful aria, in which dreams soar, improves memory, learning, and emotional well-being.

The Power of a Good Night's Sleep: Balancing Sleep and Health

Quality sleep is more than simply feeling refreshed; it is a regulator of total health, impacting everything from physical health to mental clarity and emotional resiliency. *Here are some highlights from the symphony of sleep's benefits:*

- Physical Health: Deep sleep boosts our immune system, controls blood pressure, and lowers our risk of chronic illnesses such as diabetes and heart disease. * **Mental Clarity:** REM sleep improves memory, learning, and cognitive function, keeping our thoughts sharp and focused.
- Emotional Resilience:Adequate sleep controls mood, decreases stress and anxiety and promotes a sense of well-being.
- Increased vigor:Waking up feeling refreshed and revitalized helps us to face the day with vigor and excitement.

Overcoming Obstacles: Tuning Out Sleep Disruptors

Life's melodies may sometimes become discordant sounds, interrupting our sleep symphony. But don't worry, even the most complicated scores can be harmonized:

- Addressing Medical Issues:*Certain medical issues might interfere with sleep.
- *Creating a Sleep Sanctuary: Transform your bedroom into a paradise for rest by seeing your doctor to rule out any underlying disorders and explore treatment choices.

- Practicing Relaxation Techniques: Before bed, calming activities such as reading, meditation, or deep breathing may help to quiet the mind and prepare it for sleep.
- Establishing a Regular Sleep Schedule:Go to bed and get up at regular times, including on weekends, to control your body's normal sleep-wake cycle.
- Avoiding Stimulants: Caffeine and alcohol use should be limited, particularly in the evening, since they may disturb sleep patterns.

Remember that getting enough sleep is a journey, not a destination. Be patient, try multiple strategies, and don't be afraid to seek professional assistance if sleep problems continue.

The Impact on Relationships and Well-Being Beyond the Individual Symphony

Quality sleep is more than simply a personal advantage; it influences our relationships and general well-being. We are more patient, empathetic, and interested in our relationships with loved ones when we are well-rested. We're better prepared to deal with life's difficulties and manage social settings with grace. Sleep serves as a link between our well-being and the peace of our communities.

Accept the Power of Rest:

Let us rewrite the story in a culture that frequently promotes activity and tiredness. Let us celebrate the power of sleep as an active investment in our health, pleasure, and well-being, rather than as a passive need. Let us transform our bedrooms into rejuvenation havens, where sleep becomes a symphony of repair and rebirth.

9

Chapter 9: Stress Management and Calming Techniques: Tools and Techniques for Maintaining Emotional Balance

L ife, with its brilliant twists and turns, may sometimes seem like an emotional rollercoaster. While exciting, the ups and downs may leave us frustrated, apprehensive, and overwhelmed. However, in this chapter, we'll explore the art of emotional landscaping, looking at tools and tactics for taming stress and creating an inner oasis of peace, particularly in later life.

Beyond the White Knuckles: Reframing the Stress Narrative in Later Life

Forget the preconceptions of elderly people who are always anxious about money, health, or family. Stress is unavoidable, but it does not have to define our lives. Let us reframe the story, seeing stress not as an adversary to be defeated, but as an unpleasant visitor we can learn to handle and graciously dismiss.

The Emotional Symphony: Understanding the Chorus and the Conductor

Consider our emotions to be a complicated symphony, with each emotion acting as a separate instrument. In this example, stress is like a loud drumming that drowns out the symphony of peace, pleasure, and satisfaction. Our objective is to raise the loudness such that the more harmonic tones rise above the din.

The Mindfulness Maestro: Taking Charge of Our Thoughts and Reactions

Mindfulness, like a skillful conductor, enables us to take control of our thoughts and behaviors, guiding them away from the discordant cacophony of stress and toward the serene symphony of serenity. *Here are some tools from the mindfulness toolbox:*

- Meditation:This practice educates our brains to examine thoughts and emotions objectively, enabling them to slip away naturally. A few minutes of meditation each day may greatly decrease stress and anxiety.
- Deep Breathing: Deep breathing stimulates the parasympathetic nervous system, which promotes relaxation and lowers stress hormones.
- Body Scan Meditation: Concentrating on physical sensations from head to toe may help us stay in the present moment and divert our attention away from mental tension.
- Gratitude Practice: Developing a grateful attitude and taking time to appreciate the wonderful things in life may help us change our attention and increase positive feelings.

Harmonizing with Harmony: Stress-Reducing Lifestyle Choices

Our everyday habits and decisions are like individual solos that contribute to the broader symphony of our well-being. *Here are some notes that accompany a stress-free melody:*

- Regular Exercise: Physical exercise releases endorphins, which work as natural mood lifters and aid in the management of stress hormones. Discover activities that you love, such as walking, swimming, or dancing.

- Healthy Diet: Nourishing our bodies with nutritious meals fuels our resilience and mental well-being. Avoid processed meals, sugar, and caffeine, all of which may aggravate stress.
- Adequate Sleep: Sleep is a soothing lullaby for our thoughts and bodies. Make excellent sleep a priority for maximum emotional and physical recovery.
- Connect with Loved Ones:Social engagement and emotional support are essential for stress management. Spend time with friends and family, express your worries, and engage in meaningful discussions.
- Participating in Hobbies: Hobbies that we like and find rewarding give us a mental break from stress and allow us to replenish our emotional batteries. Find a hobby that you like, whether it's reading, gardening, or music.

Overcoming Obstacles: When the Music Becomes Discordant

Even the most meticulously planned symphonies may be disrupted by life's unexpected sounds. If stress becomes overpowering, remember the following chords of support:

Seek Professional assistance: If stress has a substantial influence on your life, don't be afraid to seek professional assistance from a therapist or counselor. They may provide tailored assistance and coping methods.

Be a part of a Support Group: Connecting with individuals who understand your situation may be quite valuable. Sharing experiences and learning from one another may help to reduce feelings of loneliness while also providing vital insights.

Pay Attention to Progress, Not Perfection: Remember that stress management is a process, not a destination. Be kind to yourself, rejoice in minor accomplishments, and have faith in the process of learning and changing.

Keep in mind that establishing emotional balance does not imply completely removing stress. It is about cultivating the skills and fortitude needed to face life's unavoidable obstacles with grace and tranquility. We may convert our internal landscape into a refuge of tranquility by embracing mindfulness, making healthy lifestyle choices, and seeking out help when required, enabling the soothing symphony of well-being to resound throughout our lives.

Beyond the Meditation Mat: Relaxation and Emotional Well-Being Activities

we looked at how mindfulness might help you manage stress and cultivate calm. Now, let's go beyond the meditation mat to uncover a thriving symphony of activities that might promote relaxation and mental well-being, particularly at a later age. Remember that a comprehensive approach to emotional balance incorporates a wide range of melodies, enabling you to choose the harmonies that speak to your soul the most.

Nature's Symphony: Immersing in Outdoor Tranquility

Entering nature is like entering a tranquil haven. The sounds of rustling leaves, the aroma of pine needles, the warmth of the sun on your skin - these natural harmonies soothe the spirit, lowering tension and increasing emotional well-being. *Here are some ideas for enjoying nature's symphony:*

- Forest Bathing: Take in the ambiance of a woodland environment. Take slow breaths, leisurely walks, and just be present in the tranquil surroundings.
- Growing: Plant care is a grounding hobby that ties you to the land and encourages attention. Seeing fruits and vegetables develop is a satisfying experience that fosters a feeling of success and well-being.
- Birdwatching: Observing birds' vivid tunes and beautiful movements may be unexpectedly relaxing. It encourages concentration, patience, and amazement of the natural world.
- Picnics in the Park: Pack a nutritious snack basket, locate a sunny area beneath a tree, and enjoy a peaceful dinner surrounded by nature. Sharing it with family and friends gives an extra element of social connection and

delight.

Artistic Expressions: Unleashing Your Inner Creativity

Engaging in creative activities may be an effective stress-reduction and emotional expression technique. It helps you to channel your inner artist, explore your emotions, and create something beautiful as a result. *Here are some musical compositions to consider:*

- Painting or Drawing: Experiment with different colors and textures. Direct your emotions onto the canvas, resulting in a visual portrayal of your inner environment.
- Writing: Whether journaling or creating tales, writing allows for emotional expression and introspection. Putting pen to paper may assist you in processing problems and gaining fresh views.
- *Music: Learn an instrument, sing along to your favorite songs, or immerse yourself in a concert's melodies. Music has a powerful emotional influence, promoting pleasure, relaxation, and a feeling of connection.
- Dancing: Allow your body to move freely, express yourself via rhythm, and let the music lead you. Dancing is a fun method to relieve stress, increase energy, and connect with your inner child.

Mindful Movement: Gentle Activities to Connect Body and Mind

When undertaken mindfully, physical exercise may be a powerful tool for stress reduction and emotional balance. Gentle and focused movements promote body-mind connection, enabling you to move with grace and awareness. *Here are a few mindful motions to try:*

- Yoga: This ancient practice promotes flexibility, strength, and inner serenity by combining physical postures, breathing exercises, and meditation. Several moderate techniques, such as restorative yoga, are appropriate for seniors.
- Tai Chi: Tai Chi is a great mix of mindfulness and physical exercise, with its flowing, beautiful motions and concentrated breathing. It helps with

balance, coordination, and general well-being.

- Meditation While Walking: Make your everyday stroll a mindful practice. Concentrate on your body's feelings, the rhythm of your breath, and the sights and sounds around you. Walking meditation is a grounded and approachable method of practicing mindfulness in motion.
- Aqua Fitness: Gentle water movements provide a low-impact workout that is gentle on the joints. Water's buoyancy creates a sense of weightlessness, encouraging relaxation and stress reduction.

Keep in mind that there is no one-size-fits-all solution to relaxation and mental well-being.

10

Chapter 10: Discovering Your Purpose: Finding Meaning and Fulfillment Later in Life

As the chapters of life unfold, the storyline often swings from lofty goals to whispers of "what's next?" In this chapter, we'll enjoy the lively melody of later years while delving into the tremendous yearning for meaning, purpose, and satisfaction. Forget rocking rockers and empty nests; this is a voyage of reigniting passions, exploring new frontiers, and enhancing your life with contributions that reverberate from the heart of your being.

Beyond the Retirement Horizon: Redefining the Purpose Concept

Purpose isn't a prize to be won at the end of adolescence; it's a lively seed that may bloom at any age. Forget about lofty speeches and social expectations. Your mission is one-of-a-kind, an exquisite tapestry woven from your life experiences, interests, and beliefs. It's about discovering what makes your soul sing, what piques your interest, and what drives you to contribute to the world in a genuine and rewarding manner.

The Symphony of Passion: Finding Inner Harmony

Consider your goal to be a tune ready to be performed. To hear its tones, go within and explore your hobbies and interests. ***Here are some instruments to get you started:***

- Reflect on your past: What activities in prior chapters offered you delight and satisfaction? Did you like experimenting with gadgets, getting lost in tales, or interacting with others? Revisiting old interests might stimulate new thoughts and reveal latent yearning.
- Explore new frontiers: Don't let age or imagined restrictions hold you back. Try new things, attend lessons, and volunteer in various areas. You could uncover a secret aptitude for painting, a love of environmental advocacy, or a skill for teaching grandkids how to bake.
- Listen to your heart: Pay attention to what piques your interest, causes you to lose track of time, and lights a fire in your belly. These are often clues of your ultimate mission, which is only waiting to be disclosed.

Harmonizing with the World: Discovering Your Special Contribution

Your mission is a beautiful collaboration with the world around you, not a solo performance. Look beyond yourself to see how your interests and abilities may help others and make a difference in their lives. ***Here are some notes to consider:***

- Sharing your knowledge: Mentoring young people, sharing your life experiences, or teaching a skill you've perfected over the years are all examples of ways to offer your wisdom. Others may benefit much from your expertise and viewpoint.
- Involvement in your community: Volunteer your time and abilities to a cause that is important to you. Working with animals, supporting local charities, or fighting environmental problems may all have a significant effect.
- Creative endeavors: Express yourself via painting, music, writing, or any other creative activity that enables you to share your distinct voice and

thoughts with the rest of the world.

- Connections: Develop meaningful ties with friends, family, and loved ones. Strong social relationships are essential for happiness and may provide a sense of purpose and satisfaction.

Overcoming Obstacles: When the Music Becomes Discordant

The melody of life might occasionally become dissonant sounds of uneasiness, self-doubt, or failure anxiety. But keep in mind that discovering your purpose is a journey, not a destination. *Here are some chords to harmonize with for support:*

- Embrace Imperfection: Don't wait for the ideal timing or plan. Begin small, take action, and learn from your mistakes. The most rewarding adventures often start with a single step into the unknown.
- Silence the inner critic:Is that voice of doubt telling you that "you're too old" or "it's too late"? Challenge it with positive affirmations and have faith in your abilities.
- Look for inspiration:Surround yourself with tales of those who have discovered their calling later in life. Learn from their experiences, get inspiration, and understand that it is never too late to revitalize your life.
- Celebrate Progress: Notice and celebrate tiny successes, as well as moments of pleasure and delight along the path. Recognizing your progress motivates you and keeps the tune of purpose playing in your head.

Keep in mind that discovering your mission is not about obtaining fame or fortune. It's about living a life that is in line with your ideals, contributing to something greater than yourself, and waking up every day delighted to be a part of the world's symphony. The flexibility to rediscover your interests, readjust your ambitions, and create a new chapter filled with purpose and satisfaction is the beauty of later years.

connecting with like-minded

we looked at the transformational path of discovering your life's purpose later in life. The ability to interact with like-minded people is an important harmonic in this symphony of joy. Sharing the stage with individuals who share your interests, beliefs, and aspirations may improve your trip in a variety of ways:

Amplifying the Purpose Melody:

- *Collaborative inspiration: Surround yourself with others who share your hobbies, aspirations, or creative endeavors. Their energy may be infectious, boosting your ambition and pressing you ahead. Seeing their accomplishments might motivate you to pursue your own goals.
- Mutual support: When confronted with a supportive community, life's obstacles and uncertainties might seem less intimidating. Sharing experiences, providing advice, and enjoying accomplishments together builds a safety net of support and understanding.
- Co-creation and collaboration: Similar-minded people may become great collaborators by brainstorming ideas, collaborating on projects, or just sharing their distinct viewpoints. This collaborative mindset may lead to enjoyable experiences and increase the effect of your common goal.

Alignment with the World:

- *Broadening your horizons:Meeting individuals from different backgrounds and experiences may help you comprehend the world and your position in it. Sharing opinions and learning from one another may lead to personal development and a stronger feeling of community.
- Having a greater impact:When like-minded people band together, their combined energy and resources may generate a good ripple effect.

Whether you're lobbying for a cause, launching a community project, or just sharing pleasure, your combined efforts may have a far-reaching influence that goes beyond individual efforts.

How to Deal with Loneliness and Isolation: Feeling connected and respected is critical for happiness, particularly in later life. Connecting with like-minded people may help to alleviate loneliness and isolation while also building a feeling of belonging and social support. Laughter shared with others, meaningful talks, and true friendships improve your life and add to your overall pleasure and contentment.

Remember that making relationships with like-minded people is an ongoing process.*Here are some ideas for finding your tribe:*

- Join local clubs or groups: Look into organizations that cater to your interests, whether it's a reading club, an art class, a volunteer group, or a senior center with a variety of activities. Connecting with others online may be a terrific method to meet like-minded people, particularly if you are limited by geography.
- Attend events and conferences: Look for events that are linked to your hobbies or interests, where you may meet people who share your excitement.
- Give back to your community: Volunteering in your community is a great opportunity to meet new people and contribute to something useful while connecting with others who share your beliefs.
- Be friendly and open: Don't be hesitant to start up a conversation with random strangers. You may be surprised to find common interests and make unexpected connections.

Connecting with like-minded people is more than merely finding people who agree with you. It's about appreciating differences within the context of a common song of purpose. Accept the diversity of your experiences, viewpoints, and abilities. Allow the harmonic notes of connection to fill the symphony of your life, magnifying your purpose, enhancing your path, and producing a lively chorus of satisfaction in the latter chapters of your life.

58

11

Chapter 11: The Twenties and Thirties: Laying the Groundwork for a Healthy Future

L ife seems like a tornado of possibilities throughout your twenties and thirties. Career goals take flight, relationships develop, and the world beckons with limitless opportunities. But, despite the excitement, it's important to remember that these formative years are also an excellent opportunity to set the groundwork for a healthy and successful future.

This chapter explores the potential of proactive health decisions in your twenties and thirties, not as a burdensome duty, but as a powerful investment in your well-being. We'll look at practical suggestions and techniques for developing healthy habits, navigating the intricacies of nutrition and exercise, and prioritizing mental and emotional well-being, all while enjoying the unique difficulties and possibilities that come with this wonderful period of life.

The Health Symphony: Tuning in to Your Body's Rhythm

Consider your body to be a complicated musical instrument. The decisions you make - the food you feed it, the manner you exercise it, the thoughts you give it - are the notes that make up your health's symphony. You can tune this instrument throughout your twenties and thirties, producing a harmonic song that echoes through every chapter of your life.

Harmonizing with Nutritional Notes:

- Fuel for the Journey: Avoid processed and sugary foods in favor of a diet rich in healthy foods, fruits, vegetables, and lean protein. These give critical nutrients and energy to support your active lifestyle and overall health.
- Mindful Eating: Slowly chew your food and pay attention to your body's hunger signals. Avoid thoughtless snacking and emotional eating by making intentional decisions that feed both your body and mind.
- Hydration Balance: Water acts as the director of your internal symphony, ensuring that everything runs properly. To keep your body hydrated and operating effectively, avoid sugary beverages and favor water throughout the day.

Getting in Shape for Exercise:

- Discover Your Groove: Exercise does not have to be difficult. Explore your interests, whether it's dancing to your favorite music, cycling along gorgeous routes, or working out at the gym. Finding a regimen that you can keep and that provides you with delight is essential.
- Strength and endurance:Don't forget about strength training. Muscle mass not only increases your metabolism but also your bone density and general fitness. Aim for many strength training sessions each week that target all main muscle groups.
- Pay Attention to Your Body: Rest and rehabilitation are critical for injury prevention and performance enhancement. Don't overwork yourself; instead, pay attention to your body's signals and take rest days as required.

Mind and Emotional Tuning:

- Stress Management Symphony: Life may be difficult, but you have control over how you respond to it. To control stress and create inner peace, use relaxation methods such as deep breathing, meditation, or yoga.
- Sleep is Good for the Soul: Make 7-8 hours of excellent sleep a priority each night. Sleep is necessary for both physical and mental well-being because it allows your body and mind to rejuvenate and consolidate memories.
- Social Relationships: Emotional wellness requires strong social relationships. Develop your connections with friends and family, seek help when you need it, and create a community that elevates and inspires you.

Overcoming Obstacles: When the Music Becomes Discordant

Life in your twenties and thirties can be a balancing act, managing work goals, personal relationships, and the temptation to "have it all." It is inevitable to encounter difficulties and failures along the route. ***To help you navigate the discordant sounds, here are some chords of support:***

- Embrace Imperfection:Do not compare your path to the journeys of others. Concentrate on your advancement, appreciate tiny triumphs, and learn from your missteps. Remember that a healthy future is established gradually, not quickly.
- Seek Professional Help: If you are experiencing particular health conditions, mental health concerns, or trouble managing stress, don't be afraid to seek professional assistance. Doctors, therapists, and dietitians may all provide helpful advice and support.
- Make Self-Compassion a Priority:Be kind with yourself. Forgive yourself for your mistakes, appreciate your accomplishments, and treat yourself with the same love and care you would give to a loved one.

Keep in mind that creating a healthy future isn't about deprivation or rigid limitations.Making educated decisions, prioritizing your well-being, and finding pleasure in the process are all important. You can create the beginning chapters of a vibrant health narrative in your twenties and thirties, one delicious taste, mindful movement, and calm breath at a time. You may improve your health by listening to your body's rhythm and making mindful decisions.

12

Chapter 12: The 40s and 50s: Priorities and Embracing Change

The 40s and 50s were a whirling kaleidoscope of life's unfolding. Peaks in one's career collide with family obligations, aspirations simmer alongside duties, and the term "balance" takes on new meaning. This chapter isn't about surviving midlife; it's about flourishing in the middle of it all, a symphony of self-discovery performed on the strings of priorities, resilience, and the exciting embracing of change.

The Harmonious Juggling Act: Priorities and Grace

Consider life to be a multi-tiered circus show, balancing work goals, family demands, relationships, and personal well-being. What is the key? Mastering the skill of smooth, conscious balance, rather than eliminating activities. *Here are some pointers to help you perfect your juggling act:*

- Prioritize with Purpose: Not every ball requires the same amount of attention. Identify your essential values, and what is important to you, and utilize them to guide your time and energy allocation. Delegate, outsource, and accept "good enough" when it does not jeopardize your principles.
- Share and collaborate: Don't try to do it alone. When the juggling pins wobble, open communication with your spouse, family, and friends may

form a supporting network, acting as a safety net. Share duties, assign work, and share successes as a group.

- Adopt Flexibility: Life is a continuous dance, not a set pattern. Schedule flexibility may be your friend, allowing you to adjust to unanticipated situations without disrupting your peace. Be open to new experiences and possibilities, and modify your route as required.

Navigating Change's Melodies: Embracing Transformation with Open Arms

Change, once dreaded, may become a lovely song in the symphony of your forties and fifties. This is a moment to find yourself, redefine your ambitions, and let go of what no longer serves you. *Here are some chords that go well with transformational music:*

- Extreme Your Comfort Zone:** Don't be scared to push yourself beyond of your comfort zone. Explore new hobbies, take up a pastime you've always wanted to try, or go on that adventurous trip you've been thinking about. Outside of the familiar, growth thrives.
- Embrace Innovation:Your job path does not have to be straight. Pursue your interests, retrain for a new career, or start your own business. This is the moment to rework your professional story to reflect your current wants and ambitions.
- Release and revitalize:Let rid of what no longer serves you. Forgive previous expectations, let go of limiting beliefs, and allow room for new chapters to emerge. Clear up your physical and mental areas to make a place for new possibilities.

How to Overcome Discordant Notes: When the Juggling Act Fails

Even the best juggler will sometimes drop a ball. The 40s and 50s have their own set of obstacles, such as balancing professional demands, negotiating changing family relationships, and dealing with bodily changes, but remember that you are not alone. ***Here are several harmonies to help you when the song goes off-key:***

- Seek Help: Don't be afraid to ask for assistance. Communicate with friends, family, therapists, or mentors. Sharing your difficulties and responsibilities might help to ease the weight and provide new insights.
- Make Self-Care a Priority: It's not selfish; it's necessary. Invest in your well-being by engaging in things that you like, such as mindfulness techniques, exercise, time in nature, and connecting with loved ones. A revitalized spirit juggles with more vigor and elegance.
- Rejoice in Progress: Don't get too caught up in the juggling act. Celebrate your accomplishments, large and small. Recognize your perseverance, acknowledge your progress, and enjoy the splendor of this exciting time of life.

Remember that in your 40s and 50s, balancing priorities and accepting change isn't about attaining picture-perfect harmony. It's about accepting life's wonderful, messy complexity, learning to negotiate the odd lost ball, and finding pleasure in the never-ending dance of metamorphosis. This is the moment to rewrite the soundtrack of your life, one conscious decision, one accepted challenge, one act of self-compassion at a time. Accept the rhythm of change, believe in your resilience, and watch the symphony of your 40s and 50s develop with grace and brightness.

13

Chapter 13: Redefining Retirement and Living Life to the Fullest: 60s and Beyond

Retirement is a phrase that many people associate with rocking chairs and days spent watching the world go by. However, in the vivid symphony of life, the latter chapters have a much richer melody, a chorus of possibilities far bigger than ordinary rocking chairs and lazy days. The 60s and beyond are a spectacular crescendo, a time to redefine retirement, rewrite the story, and enjoy life to the fullest.

Deconstructing the Retirement Myth: Harmonizing with a New Rhythm

In the conventional sense, retirement is a fading note in the symphony of contemporary life. Forget about strict timetables and forced ends. Today's 60s and beyond are fertile ground for reinvention, a moment to let go of obsolete expectations and embrace a kaleidoscope of possibilities.

- Retirement is a journey, not an endpoint:It's a versatile environment in which to pursue interests, travel to foreign locations, give back to the community, and discover unknown territory inside yourself.
- There is no one-size-fits-all solution: Create your own retirement plan. Create a rhythm that resonates with your spirit, whether it's gradual withdrawal, a total job shift, or giving your knowledge.

- Be open to lifelong learning:Curiosity never dies. Keep your mind occupied and broaden your horizons by studying a new language, diving into a historical period, or learning a musical instrument.

Tuning Your Passions: A Vibrant Symphony of Possibilities

The 60s and beyond are a great time to let go of any pent-up passions that have been simmering on the back burner throughout your earlier chapters. Allow these melodies to take center stage, producing a symphony of satisfaction and joy:

- Follow your artistic muse:** Paint, write, sculpt, or perform music - kindle your creative fire and express yourself in ways you've always wanted to.
- Explore the world with new eyes: Explore ancient ruins, climb majestic mountains, get lost in bustling foreign markets - the world is your oyster, and there's no age limit on wanderlust. * **Give back to your community:** Share your wisdom, volunteer your skills, mentor the next generation - your experience and knowledge can be a source of inspiration and support.
- Improve your physical well-being:Participate in activities that get you moving, laughing, and feeling alive. Hiking, dancing, swimming, and gardening are all activities that may bring you delight and enjoy the advantages of an active lifestyle.

Connecting with Others: Harmonizing with the World

Life is an orchestra, and we are all instruments, our songs complementing each other's. Embrace the power of connection in your 60s and beyond, creating harmonies that vibrate with delight and meaning:

- Nurture existing relationships:** Invest in friendships, spend quality time with loved ones, and make memories that will last a lifetime. These relationships are the foundations of our happiness.

- Expand your social circle:Join groups, attend seminars, and take courses to meet new people with similar interests and hobbies. Making new relationships keeps you active and interested.
- Travel with loved ones:Plan joint excursions, discover the globe with your partners, and form even stronger ties. These shared experiences will be remembered fondly.
- *Give back to your community:Offer your time and talents to a cause that is important to you. Making a difference in the world gives you a lot of happiness and improves your connection with your surroundings.

Overcoming Obstacles: When the Music Becomes Discordant

Even in its final chapters, life's symphony is not immune to dissonant notes. Health issues, family upheaval, and loneliness may all throw shadows on an otherwise brilliant environment. Here are various chords of support to use when the music falls flat:

- Seek help and support:If you are experiencing health problems or emotional difficulties, do not be afraid to seek expert assistance. Speak with your doctor, counselor, or therapist; help is available.
- Embrace your community:Tap into your support system of friends, family, and loved ones. Their understanding and support may be a source of strength and comfort.
- Pay attention to mindfulness and self-care:Set aside time for activities that feed your mind, body, and spirit. Meditation, spending time in nature, and engaging in things that you like may help you find calm and resilience.
- Celebrate your journey: Regardless of the obstacles, recognize your progress, admire your perseverance, and rejoice in the minor successes that enrich your life.

Note that reinventing retirement and enjoying life to the fullest in your 60s and beyond isn't about perfection. It's about embracing life's dynamic melody, finding delight in the unexpected, and constantly rewriting your life's story. Allow your passions to be the leading melody, your relationships to be the harmonic chorus, and your resilience to be the steady pace.

69

14

Chapter 14: Overcoming Age-Related Obstacles: Maintaining Independence While Managing Chronic Conditions

The vivid symphony of our existence unavoidably faces crescendos of problems as the last chapters of life unfold. Age-related problems, such as chronic diseases and the need for increasing assistance, may develop, casting shadows on our journey's bright songs. However, even in the middle of these difficulties, we may learn to harmonize with resilience, traverse the terrain with elegance, and keep the lovely song of independence.

Tuning Your Body's Instrument: Managing Chronic Conditions with Proactive Care

Chronic diseases, previously considered unwanted visitors, may be blended into your life's symphony with careful treatment.

Here are some chords to consider:

- Knowledge is power: Become knowledgeable about your disease, its triggers, and management options. Consult your doctor regularly, ask questions, and take an active role in your own treatment.
- Adopt a holistic approach: Consider alternative therapies such as yoga,

meditation, or acupuncture in addition to orthodox treatments. Investigate dietary changes to see what works best for your body and overall health.

- Create a support network:Surround yourself with healthcare experts, loved ones, and support groups who are familiar with your situation. Their knowledge, understanding, and support may be helpful.
- Empower yourself with technology: Use assistive devices, medication reminders, and telehealth tools to effectively manage your disease while maintaining your freedom. Technology may be an invaluable ally in negotiating difficulties.

How to Harmonize with Independence: Autonomy Strategies

Throughout life's chapters, the longing for freedom remains a passionate symphony. *Here are some strategies to maintain your autonomy:*

- Proactive Planning:Anticipate future requirements and make well-informed judgments. Consider your living situation, financial stability, and transportation choices to guarantee your freedom as your requirements change.
- Embrace Adaptability:Life may be unpredictable. Be adaptable in your routines and everyday activities to meet your changing demands. Accept technology, delegate chores, and seek assistance when required without jeopardizing your autonomy.
- Focus on Functional Fitness:Exercise regularly to maintain strength, balance, and flexibility. Even little changes to your routine may make a huge impact on your ability to handle everyday chores and maintain your independence.
- Stay Socially Connected: Loneliness may steal your freedom silently. Develop friends, participate in social events, and give back to your community. Social relationships may help you stay active and engaged by providing emotional support.

Overcoming Discordant Notes: When Difficulties Appear Overwhelming

The process of managing chronic diseases and retaining independence may be difficult, with frustrating and uncertain times. Remember, they are normal notes in life's symphony. When the music becomes harsh, ***here are some chords to harmonize with:***

- Acknowledge your feelings:Holding on to bad emotions may be harmful. Discuss your concerns and anxieties with loved ones, a therapist, or a support group. Sharing your weight might lighten your load and open up new possibilities.
- Rejoice in minor victories:Setbacks should not discourage you. Concentrate on your progress, no matter how modest. Each step you take in managing your health or maintaining your independence should be celebrated.
- Experience self-compassion:Be kind with yourself. Accepting limits and recognizing problems does not imply giving up. Self-compassion is essential for overcoming challenges with resilience.
- Seek professional assistance: Seek expert assistance if you are experiencing emotional difficulties or managing challenging healthcare issues. Therapists, social workers, and geriatric care managers may all provide vital advice and assistance.

Remember, addressing age-related issues is not about muting your life's melodies. It's about learning to play a new version of your symphony, adjusting your pace, and accepting the backup instruments that enable you to continue crafting the music of your life. You may traverse these problems with grace, keeping the rich harmonies of your life in its final chapters, provided you practice proactive care, resilience, and a focus on maintaining independence.

Living in Balance: Practical Advice and Resources for Managing Chronic Conditions

Later chapters of life are often enhanced by knowledge and experience, but they may also offer new obstacles in the shape of chronic diseases. Whether it's diabetes, arthritis, heart disease, or any other chronic health condition, maintaining the song of well-being playing strong requires proactive management and astute inventiveness. ***Here's a guide to handling certain chronic diseases, along with helpful hints, nutritional suggestions, and assistive technology options:***

Diabetes:

- Activity Routines: Aim for 150 minutes per week of moderate-intensity activity such as brisk walking, swimming, or cycling. For encouragement and support, consider joining a diabetes-friendly fitness club.
- Dietary Guidelines: Make whole foods like fruits, veggies, and lean protein a priority. Limit your intake of processed meals, fizzy drinks, and saturated fat. For individualized nutritional advice, see a qualified nutritionist.
- Assistive Technology:Continuous glucose monitoring devices can check blood sugar levels in real-time, allowing you to make more educated food and physical activity choices. Insulin pumps provide accurate insulin administration, making medication management easier.

Arthritis:

- Exercise Routines: Low-impact workouts such as water aerobics, yoga, or tai chi may help with joint flexibility and pain relief. Stretching daily is essential for preserving joint mobility.
- Dietary Recommendations: Eat anti-inflammatory foods including fatty fish, almonds, and antioxidant-rich fruits. Avoid processed meals as well as those heavy in saturated and trans fats, since they might aggravate

inflammation.

- Assistive Technology: To alleviate joint strain during everyday chores, consider employing grab bars, shower chairs, and ergonomic gadgets. Canes and walkers may help with stability and movement.

Heart Problems:

- Activity Routines: On most days of the week, aim for at least 30 minutes of moderate-intensity activity. Choose enjoyable hobbies such as gardening, dancing, or vigorous walking.
- Dietary Guidelines: Adopt a heart-healthy diet that includes plenty of fruits and vegetables, whole grains, and lean protein. Limit your consumption of saturated fat, cholesterol, and salt. For individualized nutritional recommendations, see your doctor or a licensed nutritionist.
- Aided Technology: Blood pressure and heart rate monitors may assist you in tracking your cardiovascular health and making educated lifestyle decisions. Personalized health coaching and assistance may be provided via mobile health applications.

Visual Impairment:

- Adaptive Exercises: To keep active and interested while exercising, use audio explanations. Consider guided walks or training programs created for those who have lost their eyesight.
- Dietary Recommendations:Make sure you get enough vitamins A, C, and E, which are vital for eye health. Increase your intake of fruits, vegetables, and leafy greens.
- Assistive Technology: Use magnifying glasses, screen readers, and voice-activated technologies to help you manage everyday tasks more independently. Consider using audio books, audiobooks, and specialized technologies to get knowledge and amusement.

Hearing Impairment:

- Social Engagement: Stay connected with friends and family in public places by using video calls, group activities, and assistive listening devices. Isolation may be alleviated by active engagement in social activities.
- Dietary Recommendations: Eat a nutritious diet rich in vitamins and minerals that are important for hearing health. Specific dietary suggestions should be sought from your doctor or a qualified nutritionist.
- Aided Technology: Invest in hearing aids that are appropriate for your hearing requirements and preferences. Consider closed captioning equipment for TV and movies, as well as amplification devices for phone calls and chats in loud surroundings.

Keep in mind that these are merely beginning points. Consult your healthcare professional for particular advice on managing your chronic illness. They may suggest additional resources, specialized fitness routines, and food regimens that are suited to your specific requirements and interests.

Alternative Resources:

National Institutes of Health (NIH): Offers comprehensive information on various chronic conditions and treatment options.

Centers for Disease Control and Prevention (CDC):Provides resources and guidelines for managing chronic conditions and maintaining healthy lifestyle habits.

Harmonizing with Support: The Influence of Social Support in Later Life

The tapestry of life is stitched with bright strands of experience, knowledge, and perseverance. However, navigating this terrain, especially when dealing with chronic diseases or other age-related issues, often needs the strength and comfort of a strong support network. Building a strong community around you - a chorus of support resonating with the voices of family, friends, healthcare experts, and community resources - becomes an important tune in the symphony of well-being.

Family and Friends: The Harmonious Inner Circle

Our loved ones are the most intimate chords in our support network, their melodies ringing with profound comprehension and undying care. Sharing hardships with family and friends may help to ease the strain, while their support and company can provide pleasure and significance to everyday life.

- Participate in Shared Activities:Plan shared activities such as walks in nature, game evenings, or just leisurely discussions to build your friendships and provide emotional shelter.
- Seek Open Communication: Don't be afraid to communicate your difficulties and wants. Open communication with family and friends helps them to adjust their support while also building trust and connection.
- Embrace Their Roles: Recognize each loved one's distinct contributions. A kid may give technical assistance, a friend may lend a sympathetic ear, and a spouse or partner may share daily activities and obligations.

Healthcare Professionals: Symphony of Health Experts

Doctors, nurses, therapists, and other healthcare professionals are helpful navigators on the path to chronic illness management. Their knowledge serves as an important contrast to the song of your well-being.

- Proactive Communication:Consult your healthcare team regularly, freely sharing your problems and asking questions. This collaboration encourages educated decision-making and provides the best possible treatment.
- Seek Diverse Expertise: Depending on your unique requirements, consider partnering with therapists, nutritionists, or experts. A multidisciplinary team approach may address many elements of your health and well-being.
- Utilize Telehealth Resources: Take use of the ease of telehealth consultations for continuous assistance and direction, especially if mobility is an issue.

Community Resources: Joining the Greater Chorus

Community organizations, senior centers, and support groups may provide you with a plethora of services and connections outside of your personal circle. These varied voices add to the symphony of your happiness by offering practical aid, social involvement, and a feeling of belonging.

- Explore Local Resources:Look into support groups for your disease, elder centers that provide educational programs or social activities, and volunteer opportunities that align with your interests.
- Embrace Technology:Use online forums and social media communities to connect with others facing similar challenges and share experiences in a safe and supportive environment.
- Research Assistance Programs:Look into government-funded or community-based programs that provide practical assistance with transportation, meal delivery, or housework, easing the burden and promoting independence.

Creating and cultivating a solid support network is a continuous process.It takes commitment, honest communication, and a willingness to accept the many melodies provided by loved ones, healthcare experts, and community services. Remember, this network is more than just a safety net; it's a chorus of encouragement, a source of delight, and a strong ally in managing life's problems and possibilities as it progresses.

15

Chapter 15: Speaking Up for Yourself: Navigating Healthcare Systems and Obtaining the Treatment You Require

In the latter chapters of life, the symphony of life reaches a new crescendo, often asking us to become our conductors in the intricate orchestra of healthcare. Navigating medical systems, fighting for your needs, and ensuring you get the best treatment possible might seem like trying to interpret a complex musical score written in a foreign language. But don't worry, maestro! This chapter gives you the tools you need to raise your baton, collaborate with healthcare providers, and write the tune of well-being that resonates loudest inside you.

How to Tune Your Instrument: Knowledge is Power

Equip yourself with information before leading the symphony of your health. Investigate your medical problem, treatment choices, and relevant resources. Inform yourself about drugs, possible adverse effects, and alternative remedies. Remember that information is your first tool, allowing you to ask educated questions, actively participate in decision-making, and hold healthcare personnel responsible.

Use trusted sources: Look for information from recognized medical organizations, research publications, and patient advocacy organizations. Avoid depending exclusively on anecdotes or internet forums.

Consult your doctor: Don't be afraid to ask questions, clarify doubts, and freely voice your concerns. Your doctor is an invaluable resource and collaborator in your health journey.

Think about getting second opinions: If you are unsure or have lingering concerns, seek the advice of another healthcare practitioner. This may give useful information and enable you to make educated decisions.

The Collaborative Melody: Harmonizing with Your Healthcare Team

Your healthcare team is not simply a background band; they are fellow musicians working together to create the symphony of your well-being.

- Speak out for your priorities:Express your preferences, aims, and concerns clearly. Don't be afraid to bring up lifestyle changes, alternative treatments, or possible prescription scheduling problems.
- Ask for clarification:Ask for clarification if you don't comprehend medical language or treatment plans. Your team owes you openness and should respond to your issues in a manner that you can understand.
- Get ready for appointments: Take notes, bring a list of questions with you, and keep track of any new symptoms or changes in your health. Proactive planning ensures that your issues are addressed and that the value of your consultations is maximized.

Beyond the Doctor's Office: A More Comprehensive Symphony of Resources

The symphony of healthcare goes beyond physicians and institutions. Use the following supplementary resources to boost your well-being:

- Patient advocacy groups:These organizations give essential information, support, and connections to others who are dealing with similar issues. They may also help patients navigate the healthcare system and fight for their rights.
- Community resources: Senior centers, local health departments, and social service organizations may provide transportation, food delivery, medication administration, and other practical support.
- Technology: From the comfort of your own home, online medical resources, telehealth consultations, and prescription reminder applications may help you manage your health and remain informed.

Keep in mind that advocating for oneself is a team effort.You may convert the complicated melodies of healthcare into a harmonious symphony of well-being by arming yourself with information, speaking effectively, and using available resources. In your health journey, you are the composer, director, and lead vocalist. Raise your voice, own your power, and compose the bright symphony of health and well-being that resonates most strongly inside you.

Message Harmonization: Communication Strategies for Healthcare Advocacy

When it comes to advocating for your needs, navigating the healthcare system may seem like orchestrating a complicated symphony. But, like any good conductor, mastering communication with your healthcare team is essential to creating a beautiful symphony of well-being. *Here are some practical tips for making your voice heard loud and clear:*

Before the Curtain Rises: Appointment Preparation

- Compose a question melody:Write down any questions you have regarding your health, treatment alternatives, possible side effects, or lifestyle changes. Prioritize the questions that are most relevant to your problems.
- Document the score: Create a chronology of your symptoms, changes in

your condition, and treatments. This helps your healthcare team see the big picture.

- Assemble your instruments:Bring any pertinent medical documents, test results, and papers about your illness. Preparing ahead of time saves time and provides for a more focused conversation.

****At Appointments, Harmonize the Conversation****

- Be an active listener: Pay careful attention to your doctor's explanations and clarify any unclear points. Don't be afraid to ask for alternate explanations or visual aids.
- Speak your mind: Openly and honestly express your issues, opinions, and objectives. To make educated choices regarding your treatment, your healthcare team depends on your input.
- Set the tempo: Don't be afraid to express your desired communication speed. Inform your doctor if you need a longer time to comprehend information or have further questions.

****After the Consultation: Maintaining Performance****

- Clarify the tune: If you come across medical jargon that you don't understand, ask for simpler explanations or printed resources. Knowledge enables you to make educated decisions.
- Take notes and record conversations: This is particularly important for recalling facts and monitoring progress in complicated medical situations.
- Proactive communication: Don't wait until your next visit to express your concerns. If you notice any new symptoms, or side effects, or have any queries between appointments, contact your doctor.

Keep in mind that communication is a two-way street.It is critical to openly communicate your problems, understand your doctor's point of view, and collaborate toward common objectives to have a pleasant healthcare experience. By adopting these communication tactics, you can turn the discordant notes of healthcare complexity into a beautiful symphony of well-being, taking confident and clear charge of your health path.

Embracing Self-Care and Emotional Well-Being in Healthcare Navigation

Navigating the complicated terrain of healthcare, especially at a later age, may seem like orchestrating a complex symphony. While learning communication tactics and speaking for your needs are important instruments in this symphony, one tune that sometimes goes unnoticed is the fundamental harmony of self-care and emotional well-being. ignoring your well-being may generate discordant notes in your health journey, just as ignoring a single instrument can throw the whole concert off tune.

Tuning the Inner Instruments: Making Self-Care a Priority

In this perspective, self-care extends beyond luxurious bubble baths and spa days. It is the attentive care of your physical, emotional, and spiritual needs, ensuring they are in tune with the melodies of your healthcare journey.

- Nurture your body:Make proper sleep, nutritional food, and frequent physical exercise a priority, even if it's as simple as light walks or chair yoga. Your body is the vehicle through which you experience life, and its health is the cornerstone of your overall health.
- Nourish your mind:Do something you like, such as reading, art, spending time outside, or interacting with loved ones. Mental stimulation and delight are necessary for emotional resilience and dealing with difficult medical conditions.
- Tend to your spirit: Meditation, mindfulness techniques, and connecting with your religion may all help you find inner calm and strength. Beyond disease, finding meaning and purpose may be a great source of drive and optimism.

Harmonizing Emotions: Recognizing and Addressing Emotional Needs

Navigating healthcare may be an emotional rollercoaster of anxiety, uncertainty, irritation, and even fury. Ignoring these feelings merely exacerbates their disagreement. Instead, accept them as natural melodies along the way:

- Allow yourself to feel: Repressing emotions is unhelpful. Recognize your emotions, whether by writing, talking to a therapist, or confiding in loved ones.
- Seek emotional help:Do not be afraid to seek emotional assistance from family, friends, support groups, or mental health experts. Sharing your personal weight may relieve stress and give essential assistance.
- Construct constructive coping mechanisms: Determine good stress and anxiety management techniques, such as deep breathing exercises, mindfulness practices, or indulging in relaxing hobbies.

Integrating Self-Care and Healthcare Navigation

Self-care and emotional well-being are not frills; they are essential tools for overcoming healthcare issues. Here's how to make them work with your medical journey:

- Schedule self-care activities: Schedule self-care routines as seriously as doctor's visits. Schedule time in your calendar for activities that will feed your mind, body, and soul.
- Express your emotional needs:Don't be afraid to talk to your healthcare staff about your emotional condition. They may give information and assistance that are suited to your individual needs.
- Look for inspiration in others: Look for examples of people who have effectively included self-care and emotional well-being into their healthcare journeys. Their experiences may provide useful insights and inspiration.

Remember that self-care and emotional well-being are not diversions from healthcare; rather, they are necessary complements.Prioritizing your physical, mental, and spiritual needs creates a symphony of well-being that enables you to overcome healthcare problems with perseverance, optimism, and pleasure. You are the composer, director, and lead vocalist in this orchestra, not simply a patient. Don't ignore the instruments inside you; harmonize them with your healthcare journey to create a beautiful song of well-being that will resound throughout the chapters of your life.

16

Chapter 16: Fostering Connection and Inclusivity in Age-Friendly Communities

The last chapters of life's symphony often find us yearning for deeper connection and a stronger feeling of belonging. The music of happiness is particularly loud in dynamic communities that welcome people of all ages, weaving threads of support, inclusion, and purpose into the fabric of daily life. In this chapter, we'll look at the potential of developing age-friendly communities, places where older folks' bright spirits blend with the energy of their younger counterparts, producing a symphony of lively inclusion.

Tuning the Orchestra: Creating an Age-Friendly Neighborhood

An age-friendly community is more than just a haven for the elderly; it's a symphony of inclusion in which all people, regardless of age, may thrive. It's a landscape where walkways vibrate with the energy of interaction and shared purpose, transit alternatives dance to the beat of convenience, and public spaces hum with the energy of interaction and shared purpose.

- Accessibility is the foundation: Buildings and public places should be planned with everyone in mind, with ramps, elevators, larger entrances, and well-lit walkways providing ease of access. Transportation choices should accommodate varied mobility levels while being inexpensive and dependable.

- The pulse is social connection: Community centers, parks, and libraries should be active social gathering places, with shared activities, recreational facilities, and chances for intergenerational exchange. Social activities and events may help to bridge the generational divide by building connections and a feeling of belonging.
- The important tools are purpose and engagement: Age-friendly communities provide opportunities for older persons to share their knowledge and skills. Volunteering, mentorship programs, and intergenerational initiatives may help them channel their abilities and interests, building a feeling of purpose and communal worth.
- Technology adds to the melody:Digital literacy classes, easily accessible technology centers, and readily available tech assistance may help older individuals navigate the digital environment, bridge generational differences, and remain connected with their loved ones.

Unifying Voices: Creating an Age-Friendly Community Together

Creating an age-friendly community is not a solitary act; it is a collaborative symphony in which every voice counts. *Individuals and groups may help the symphony in the following ways:*

- Individuals: Include everyone in your everyday encounters. Help others, start discussions with individuals of all ages, and combat ageist assumptions in your network.
- Businesses: Make your stores, restaurants, and services open to the public. Provide elder discounts, age-friendly signs and furnishings, and intergenerational communication training for your personnel.
- Organizations: Advocate for age-friendly legislation, host intergenerational activities, and provide programming that meets the needs of all residents. Collaborate with local companies and community organizations to increase your influence.
- Government: Pass laws encouraging accessibility, age-inclusive housing,

and inexpensive transit choices. Invest in community centers, recreational facilities, and intergenerational programming.

Overcoming Discordant Notes: Addressing Age-Friendly Community Challenges

Creating an age-friendly community is not without its difficulties. *Here are some dissonant sounds that need to be balanced:*

- Ageism and social isolation:Use education, awareness campaigns, and facilitated encounters to combat ageist assumptions and actively support intergenerational ties.
- Limited accessibility and mobility: Advocate for accessible infrastructure, dependable transit, and adaptive housing solutions to ensure that everyone has the opportunity to participate in community life.
- Digital divide: Bridge the digital divide by providing technology literacy classes, making technology accessible, and fostering intergenerational tech assistance.
- Lack of resources and financing: Look for partnerships and community funding possibilities, as well as campaign for government assistance, to secure appropriate resources for age-friendly projects.

Remember that creating an age-friendly community is a continual process. It takes teamwork, dedication, and a never-ending effort to balance the demands of all inhabitants. We can build dynamic environments where the melodies of life echo with pleasure, purpose, and well-being for everyone by embracing inclusion, promoting connection, and empowering persons of all ages.

17

Conclusion:Aging with Grace and Gratitude: Appreciating Every Decade's Gift

Time guides us through the movements of life's symphony, much like a good conductor. The speed changes, and the melodies vary, yet the music's beauty persists with each passing decade. To age gracefully, one must not resist wrinkles or dismiss slowing notes; rather, one must dance with the beat, welcome shifting harmonies, and uncover the unique joy of each movement.

The Gratitude Gift: Gratitude is the first instrument we choose. It enables us to appreciate the richness of the decades we've already lived through, from the ecstatic crescendos of youthful laughing to the calm contemplations of knowledge gained. We learn to treasure the sun-kissed memories and the songs of love and friendship that continue to ring in our ears.

The Power of Acceptance: Acceptance becomes the song that leads us through the inevitable transformations of life. We accept the fading of youth's vivid tones and the slowing of our bodies' speed. But there is a secret beauty inside this acceptance: the room to uncover a deeper strength, a calm resilience that sprouts from the knowledge of innumerable seasons.

The Purpose Symphony: We alter the score when the beat changes. Purpose grows from the pursuit of aspirations as a child to the adult desire to leave a legacy. We mentor, share, and plant seeds of hope in future generations. Every act of kindness, every lesson gained, contributes to the symphony of a well-lived life.

The Power of Connection: Our symphony's chords do not resonate in solitude. We become friends with other travelers, exchanging tales, laughter, and tears. We learn from their songs, which enhance our own with the harmonies of shared experience. We learn from these linkages that age is not a solitary performance, but rather a dynamic ensemble, with each voice and instrument adding to the overall richness.

The Encore Is Here: As a result, we have arrived at the current moment, which is not the conclusion, but rather the prelude to the encore. We return to the stage with hearts full of appreciation, bodies receptive to change, and spirits bursting with purpose. We play with a deeper resonance this time, understanding that each note, and each sensation is a wonderful gift to be treasured, shared, and celebrated.

So let us lift our voices and instruments to the symphony of age. Let us play with elegance, appreciation, and the unwavering confidence that every decade, every note has the potential to become a masterpiece. Aging, on the other hand, is a symphony of development, a monument to the eternal beauty of a well-played life.